COUGH

UNDERSTANDING THE MESSAGE THE BODY IS SENDING THROUGH COUGH

DR. J. SIMON

Contents

INTRODUCTION

The reflexive action of coughing helps clear the airways of allergens, mucus, and foreign objects. It's the body's way of saying, "Hey, something's not quite right in the respiratory department!" The cough is your body's superhero attempt to keep the airways open and clear, regardless of the cause a bothersome cold, allergies, or even just a tickle in your throat. Thus, acknowledge your body for doing what it does best the next time you cough.

CHAPTER ONE

Definition and Overview of Cough

A cough is a protective reflex action that involves the rapid expulsion of air from the lungs to clear the throat and respiratory passages of irritants, mucus, or foreign substances. It's like the body's built-in alarm system, signaling that something needs attention in the respiratory system.

Coughs can be classified into different types, such as dry or productive (with the production of mucus or phlegm). They can be caused by various factors, including infections, allergies, irritants, or underlying medical conditions. While most coughs are temporary and self-limiting, persistent or severe coughing may indicate an underlying health issue that requires medical attention.

It's important to note that a cough itself is not a disease but rather a symptom of an underlying condition. Treatment usually focuses on addressing the root cause, whether it's a viral infection, allergies, or other respiratory issues. Over-the-counter cough suppressants or expectorants may be used to alleviate symptoms, but consulting with a healthcare professional is advisable for a proper diagnosis and guidance on the most suitable treatment.

Importance of Cough as a Protective Mechanism

Think of a cough as your body's superhero when it comes to respiratory defense! It plays a crucial role in protecting your airways and lungs from potential threats. Here's why it's such a vital protective mechanism:

Clearing Irritants: Coughing helps expel irritants, such as dust, smoke, or pollutants, from the respiratory system. It's like a quick and forceful eviction notice for anything that shouldn't be hanging around in your airways.

Removing Excess Mucus: When your body produces extra mucus in response to an infection or irritation, a cough comes in handy to get rid of that gooey stuff. It prevents mucus from building up and causing congestion.

Preventing Infections: Coughing is a defense mechanism against infections. By expelling infectious agents through coughing, your body tries to avoid letting them settle in and cause trouble.

Maintaining Airway Openness: A good cough helps keep your airways clear and open. This is especially important in preventing respiratory distress and ensuring that oxygen can flow freely to your lungs.

Alerting to Issues: Persistent or unusual coughs can signal underlying health issues. It's like your body's way of raising a flag to say, "Hey, pay attention, something might be going on here that needs checking."

So, the next time you find yourself in a coughing fit, remember that it's your body's way of working tirelessly to keep your respiratory system in top-notch shape!

Here are some common ones:

Coughing Means You're Contagious: While it's true that some contagious illnesses come with coughing, not every cough is a sign of an infectious disease. Allergies, irritants, or even just a tickle in your throat can trigger a cough.

Suppressing a Cough Is Always Bad: While coughing is a protective mechanism, there are times when suppressing it is necessary, like when you're in a meeting or trying to catch some much-needed sleep. It's about finding a balance—sometimes you need to let it out, and other times, a cough suppressant can be your ally.

All Coughs Require Antibiotics: Nope, not true. Antibiotics are effective against bacterial infections, not viral ones, which are often the cause of common colds and coughs. So, popping antibiotics for every cough won't necessarily do the trick.

Only Sick People Cough: Sure, illnesses can trigger coughs, but they're not the only culprits.

Environmental factors, allergies, or even a spicy meal can lead to a bout of coughing. It doesn't always mean you're coming down with something.

Cough Drops Cure Coughs: Hate to burst the soothing bubble, but cough drops might provide temporary relief by soothing your throat, but they don't cure the underlying cause of the cough. They're more like the sidekicks, not the superheroes.

Remember, not every cough is created equal, and understanding the root cause is key to addressing it properly. If in doubt, a chat with a healthcare professional can help clear up any misconceptions!

Let's break down the anatomy of a cough – it's like a symphony of respiratory movements working together:

Irritation or Trigger: The overture begins when something irritates your airways. It could be anything from dust particles and allergens to mucus or an invading virus. This irritation activates the body's cough reflex.

Deep Breath (Inhalation): As the first note, you take a deep breath. Your diaphragm contracts, and your chest muscles expand, drawing in air. This sets the stage for the upcoming performance.

Closure of the Glottis: Now, the glottis, the part of your larynx containing the vocal cords, snaps shut. This closure builds up pressure in your chest.

Rapid Opening of the Glottis: The glottis then opens quickly, creating a rush of air. This burst of air is the powerhouse behind the forceful expulsion that follows.

Expulsion of Air: The vocal cords snap open, and the rushing air clears the irritant or mucus from your airways. This explosive exit is the climax of the coughing symphony.

Sound Production: Depending on the force and speed of the air leaving your lungs, you may produce different sounds – from a gentle throat clearing to a hearty cough.

Relaxation: After the crescendo, your respiratory muscles relax, and you return to a calm state, awaiting the next potential trigger.

This entire process is a coordinated effort involving your respiratory muscles, diaphragm, vocal cords, and the intricate network of air passages. It's like a well-choreographed dance to keep your airways clear and your respiratory system in harmony.

Common Causes of Cough

Here are some common causes that might trigger a coughing performance:

Infections: Viral infections like the common cold or flu are classic instigators. Bacterial infections, such as bronchitis or pneumonia, can also lead to persistent coughing.

Allergies: Pollen, pet dander, dust mites—oh my! Allergic reactions can cause your immune system to go into overdrive, leading to a cough as your body tries to expel irritants.

Irritants: Smoke, air pollution, strong odors, or even chemical fumes can tickle your airways and prompt a coughing fit.

Gastroesophageal Reflux Disease (GERD): When stomach acid flows back into the esophagus, it can irritate the throat and trigger coughing. It's like an unwanted acid reflux encore.

Postnasal Drip: Excess mucus dripping down the back of your throat can be a persistent cough culprit, often associated with allergies or sinus infections.

Asthma: Wheezing, shortness of breath, and coughing can be signs of asthma, where the airways become inflamed and narrowed.

Medications: Some medications, especially ACE inhibitors used to treat high blood pressure, can cause a persistent cough as a side effect.

Environmental Factors: Changes in humidity, cold air, or exposure to respiratory irritants like mold can provoke coughing.

Chronic Conditions: Chronic obstructive pulmonary disease (COPD), bronchiectasis, or interstitial lung diseases can result in long-term coughing.

Smoking: Lighting up can not only damage your lungs but also lead to a chronic cough. It's like paying the price for a smoky performance.

Remember, a cough is often a symptom, not the main act. Identifying and addressing the underlying cause is key to finding relief and restoring peace to your respiratory theater!

Types of Cough

Coughs come in different flavors, each with its own distinct characteristics. Here are some types of coughs you might encounter:

Dry Cough (Non-productive): This cough is like a solo act—no mucus or phlegm is produced. It can be caused by irritants, allergies, or viral infections.

Wet Cough (Productive): This one's all about the phlegm. A wet cough is productive, helping to clear mucus from the airways. It's often associated with respiratory infections.

Chronic Cough: Lasting more than eight weeks, a chronic cough might indicate an underlying health issue, such as asthma, GERD, or even medication side effects.

Barking Cough: Typically seen in children, a barking cough can be a sign of croup—a viral infection affecting the upper airways.

Whooping Cough (Pertussis): This highly contagious bacterial infection causes intense bouts of coughing, often followed by a "whooping" sound when inhaling.

Nighttime Cough: Coughing that worsens at night can be linked to various factors, including postnasal drip, asthma, or GERD.

Allergic Cough: Triggered by allergens like pollen, dust, or pet dander, this cough is your body's allergic response in action.

Psychogenic Cough: Sometimes, coughing can be a habit or a response to stress, anxiety, or other psychological factors. It's like your mind playing a tune for your respiratory system.

CHAPTER TWO

Smoker's Cough: A persistent cough seen in smokers, often accompanied by increased mucus production. It's your body's way of protesting against the smoke show.

Exercise-Induced Cough: Physical activity can trigger coughing, especially in cold or dry conditions. It's like your lungs expressing their opinions on the workout.

Remember, identifying the type of cough can provide clues about its underlying cause, guiding you toward the most effective treatment or management strategy.

Coughs come with their own set of signals and symptoms, often providing clues about what might be going on in your respiratory system. Here are some common signs and symptoms associated with coughs:

Sore Throat: Coughing can irritate the throat, leading to soreness and discomfort.

Hoarseness: Persistent coughing may affect the vocal cords, resulting in a hoarse or raspy voice.

Shortness of Breath: Intense or prolonged coughing spells can leave you feeling breathless.

Chest Pain: The muscles involved in coughing are closely tied to the chest wall. Frequent and forceful coughing can cause chest discomfort or pain.

Wheezing: In conditions like asthma, coughing may be accompanied by a high-pitched whistling sound while breathing.

Fever: If your cough is due to an infection, fever might be present as your body fights off the invading pathogens.

Fatigue: Constant coughing can be physically draining, leading to fatigue and tiredness.

Runny or Stuffy Nose: Coughs associated with colds or respiratory infections often come with nasal symptoms.

Headache: The strain from persistent coughing can contribute to headaches.

Phlegm or Mucus Production: A productive cough may be accompanied by the expulsion of mucus or phlegm from the airways.

Nighttime Worsening: Coughs often intensify at night, disrupting sleep and causing discomfort.

Dizziness: Prolonged coughing episodes can sometimes lead to dizziness or lightheadedness.

Remember, these symptoms can vary depending on the underlying cause of the cough. If you're experiencing persistent or severe symptoms, it's a good idea to consult with a healthcare professional for a proper diagnosis and guidance on the most appropriate treatment.

Assessment and Diagnosis

Diagnosing and evaluating a cough involves a systematic approach to uncover its underlying cause. Here's a glimpse into the process:

Medical History: Your healthcare provider will start by asking about your medical history, including the duration and nature of the cough, any associated symptoms, and factors that worsen or alleviate it.

Physical Examination: A thorough physical examination allows the healthcare professional to assess your overall health and may include checking for signs such as chest sounds, nasal congestion, or throat irritation.

Chest X-ray: This imaging test provides a detailed view of your lungs and can help identify issues such as pneumonia, bronchitis, or lung infections.

Pulmonary Function Tests: These tests measure how well your lungs are functioning and can help identify conditions like asthma or chronic obstructive pulmonary disease (COPD).

Blood Tests: A blood sample may be taken to check for signs of infection or other systemic conditions.

Sputum Culture: If you have a productive cough, analyzing a sample of the mucus or phlegm can help identify the specific type of bacteria causing an infection.

CT Scan or MRI: In certain cases, more detailed imaging may be needed to get a closer look at the structures in the chest.

Bronchoscopy: This involves using a thin, flexible tube with a camera to examine the airways and collect samples if needed.

Allergy Testing: If allergies are suspected, tests may be conducted to identify specific allergens triggering the cough.

Acid Reflux Evaluation: In cases of suspected gastroesophageal reflux disease (GERD), tests such as pH monitoring may be performed to assess acid levels in the esophagus.

The diagnostic process aims to uncover the root cause of the cough, whether it's related to infections, allergies, respiratory conditions, or other factors. Once a diagnosis is made, appropriate treatment and management strategies can be recommended to address the specific issue. Consulting with a healthcare professional ensures a comprehensive evaluation tailored to your individual case.

Methods of Treatment

Treating a cough involves addressing the underlying cause and providing relief from symptoms. Here are some common approaches:

Self-Care and Lifestyle Modifications:

Stay hydrated: Drink plenty of fluids to help thin mucus and soothe the throat.

Use a humidifier: Moist air can ease irritation in the respiratory tract.

Avoid irritants: Steer clear of smoke, strong odors, and other respiratory irritants.

Over-the-Counter Medications:

Cough suppressants: These can help reduce the urge to cough, particularly in the case of dry or irritating coughs.

Expectorants: Designed to loosen and thin mucus, making it easier to expel.

Antihistamines: Useful for allergic coughs by blocking histamine, which contributes to allergy symptoms.

Prescription Medications:

Antibiotics: If the cough is caused by a bacterial infection, antibiotics may be prescribed.

Corticosteroids: Inhaled or oral steroids may be recommended for conditions like asthma or chronic bronchitis.

Bronchodilators:

These medications help open the airways and are commonly used in conditions like asthma or chronic obstructive pulmonary disease (COPD).

Allergy Medications:

For coughs related to allergies, antihistamines or nasal corticosteroids may be prescribed.

Lifestyle Changes:

Quit smoking: If you smoke, quitting can significantly improve respiratory health and reduce coughing.

Weight management: Losing excess weight can alleviate symptoms in conditions like sleep apnea, which may contribute to nighttime coughing.

Speech Therapy:

For persistent coughs due to vocal cord dysfunction or habit cough, speech therapy may be beneficial.

Handling of Concomitant Disorders:

Managing conditions such as GERD, asthma, or chronic respiratory diseases is essential to control associated coughing.

It's crucial to consult with a healthcare professional for an accurate diagnosis and personalized treatment plan. If a cough persists, worsens, or is accompanied by concerning symptoms, seeking medical advice ensures proper evaluation and appropriate management.

Home Remedies and Self-Care

When it comes to tackling a cough, your home is like a treasure trove of remedies. Here are some self-care tips and home remedies to ease that nagging cough:

Hydration is Key:

Drink plenty of water, herbal teas, or warm broths. Staying hydrated helps keep your throat moist and can soothe irritation.

Humidify Your Space:

Use a humidifier to add moisture to the air, especially in dry environments. This can be particularly helpful at bedtime.

Honey and Warm Tea:

Mix a teaspoon of honey into warm herbal tea. Honey can help soothe your throat, and herbal teas like chamomile or peppermint may have additional calming effects.

Gargle with Salt Water:

A classic remedy! Mix a teaspoon of salt into warm water and gargle several times a day. It can help reduce throat irritation.

Steam Inhalation:

Inhaling steam can help moisten your airways. Lean over a bowl of hot water, cover your head with a towel, and breathe in the steam. Be cautious with hot water to avoid burns.

Elevate Your Head:

Prop yourself up with extra pillows while sleeping to minimize postnasal drip and reduce nighttime coughing.

Throat Lozenges or Hard Candy:

Sucking on throat lozenges or hard candy can increase saliva production, which helps keep your throat moist and may alleviate coughing.

Avoid Irritants:

Steer clear of smoke and other environmental irritants. If possible, create a smoke-free zone around you.

Rest and Relaxation:

Ensure you get plenty of rest to help your body recover. Stress can exacerbate coughing, so relaxation techniques may also be beneficial.

Warm Salt Compress:

Soak a cloth in warm saltwater, wring it out, and place it on your chest. It can provide comfort and may help with cough associated with chest congestion.

CHAPTER THREE

Stay Warm:

Keep yourself warm, especially during colder weather. This can prevent your airways from constricting.

Coping Mechanisms and Emotional Health

Dealing with a persistent cough can be physically and emotionally challenging. Here are some coping strategies to help you navigate through it and maintain emotional well-being:

Patience and Acceptance:

Understand that a cough is often a symptom that takes time to resolve. Patience and acceptance of the situation can go a long way in reducing stress.

Seek Support:

Share your concerns and feelings with friends, family, or a healthcare professional. Having a support system can provide emotional relief and practical assistance.

Mindful Breathing and Relaxation Techniques:

Engage in mindful breathing exercises or relaxation techniques to manage stress and anxiety. Deep, slow breaths can also help soothe your respiratory system.

Distraction Techniques:

Distract yourself with activities you enjoy. Whether it's reading, watching a movie, or listening to music, finding moments of joy can positively impact your emotional well-being.

Adjust Expectations:

Modify your daily expectations and schedule based on your energy levels. Give yourself permission to take breaks and rest when needed.

Stay Informed:

Understand the cause of your cough and the treatment plan. Knowledge can empower you and alleviate anxiety about the unknown.

Stay Connected:

Even if you're not feeling your best, maintaining social connections can provide emotional support and prevent feelings of isolation.

Practice Self-Compassion:

Be kind to yourself. Recognize that coughing is a temporary symptom and not a reflection of your overall well-being.

Mind-Body Practices:

Engage in activities like yoga or tai chi that combine physical movement with mindfulness.

These practices can promote relaxation and overall well-being.

Professional Support:

If your cough is causing significant distress, consider seeking the help of a mental health professional. They can provide coping strategies and support for managing emotional challenges.

Red Flags and When to Seek Medical Attention

While most coughs are harmless and often resolve on their own, certain red flags indicate the need for prompt medical attention. Here are some signs that it's time to reach out to a healthcare professional:

Persistent Cough:

If your cough persists for more than three weeks, especially if it's worsening, it's essential to consult a healthcare provider.

Severe or Worsening Symptoms:

If your cough is accompanied by severe symptoms such as chest pain, difficulty breathing, or persistent high fever, seek medical attention promptly.

Coughing up Blood:

Coughing up blood (hemoptysis) is a serious symptom that requires immediate medical evaluation. It may indicate issues such as lung infection, injury, or even lung cancer.

Sudden Onset of Cough in a Smoker:

If you're a smoker and experience a new or different cough, it's crucial to get checked, as it could be a sign of a serious respiratory condition.

Cough in Children:

For parents, if your child has a persistent cough, difficulty breathing, or shows signs of dehydration, it's important to seek medical attention.

Wheezing or Shortness of Breath:

Persistent wheezing or shortness of breath associated with a cough may indicate conditions like asthma or bronchitis that require medical evaluation.

Cough After Travel:

If you've recently traveled and develop a cough, especially if you've been to areas with infectious diseases, it's important to seek medical attention to rule out potential infections.

Underlying Health Conditions:

If you have pre-existing conditions like asthma, COPD, or immunosuppression, a persistent cough may indicate a need for medical assessment.

Unexplained Weight Loss:

If you're experiencing unexplained weight loss along with a persistent cough, it could be a sign of an underlying health issue that requires investigation.

Cough in Older Adults:

Older adults may be at higher risk of complications from respiratory infections. If an elderly person develops a cough, especially with confusion or other concerning symptoms, seeking medical attention is important.

Cough in Special Populations

Certain populations, such as children, pregnant individuals, and older adults, may experience cough differently. Here's a brief overview of how cough can affect these special groups:

Children:

Common Causes: Children often experience coughs due to viral infections, allergies, or exposure to environmental irritants.

Concerns: Croup, a viral infection causing a barking cough, is common in younger children. Persistent or severe coughs in children should be evaluated by a healthcare professional.

Treatment: Cough medications for children should be used cautiously, following pediatrician recommendations. Humidifiers and maintaining hydration can be beneficial.

Pregnant Individuals:

Common Causes: Pregnancy can make individuals more susceptible to respiratory infections due to changes in the immune system.

Concerns: Coughs during pregnancy can cause discomfort, and certain medications may need to be avoided. It's crucial to consult with a healthcare provider for safe treatment options.

Treatment: Non-pharmacological approaches, such as humidifiers, hydration, and elevating the head during sleep, can provide relief. Pregnant individuals should consult their healthcare provider before taking any medications.

Older Adults:

Common Causes: Seniors may be more prone to respiratory infections, and coughs in this population may be related to underlying health conditions such as COPD or heart failure.

Concerns: Older adults may have weakened immune systems, making them more susceptible to complications from respiratory illnesses.

Treatment: Treatment should address the underlying cause. Older adults should receive prompt medical attention for persistent or severe coughs.

Individuals with Chronic Conditions:

Common Causes: Those with chronic conditions like asthma, COPD, or immunosuppression may experience coughs related to their underlying health issues.

Concerns: Coughs in these populations may signal exacerbations of their chronic conditions, requiring careful management.

Treatment: Treatment should be tailored to address the specific chronic condition and may involve adjustments to existing medications or additional therapies.

Conclusion

While it's often just a passing annoyance, a cough can sometimes be a subtle signal from your body that something needs attention. From dry coughs to the productive ones, the barking coughs of childhood to the persistent ones in adulthood, each has its own story.

Understanding the causes, seeking appropriate medical attention when needed, and employing self-care strategies can turn the coughing symphony into a brief solo performance. Whether it's a result of a common cold, allergies, or a more complex respiratory condition, your body's coughing reflex is a guardian of your airways, keeping them clear and functioning.

So, next time you find yourself in a coughing fit, remember to be kind to your respiratory system. Hydrate, rest, and if needed, seek the guidance of a healthcare professional to ensure a proper diagnosis and treatment plan.

THE END

www.ingramcontent.com/pod-product-compliance
Lightning Source LLC
Chambersburg PA
CBHW050705250726
48662CB00002B/859